CELL MATES

BY
BRYAN Calhoun

EDITED
BY
TERESA H. KINSFATHER

INDEX

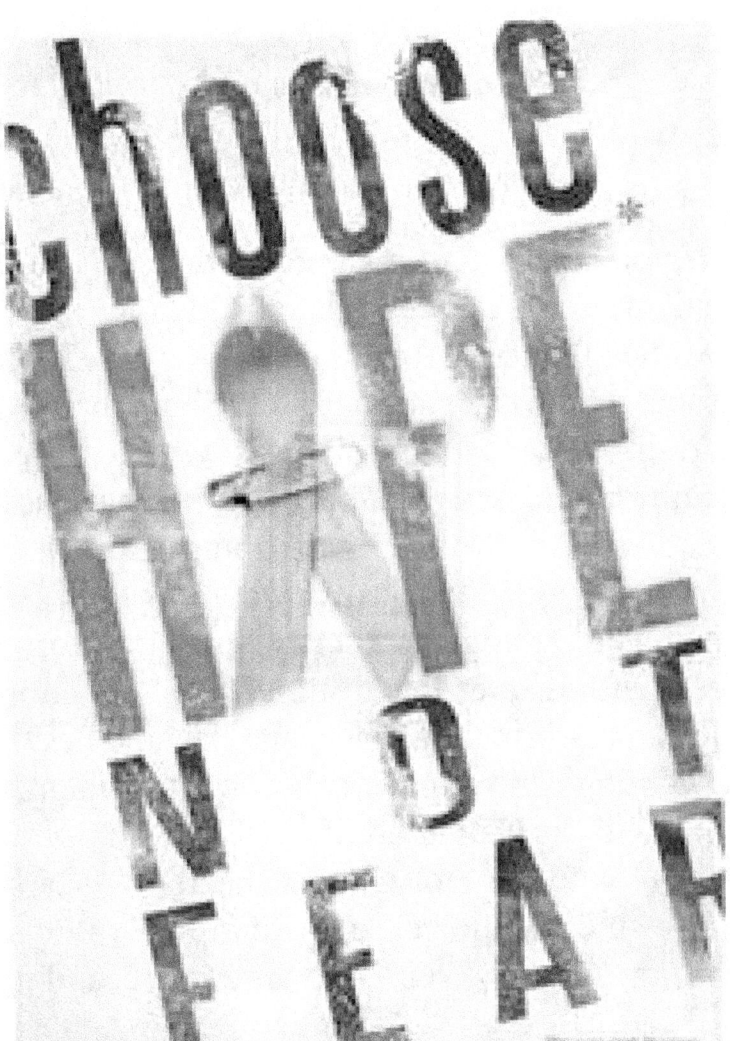

choose
HOPE*
NOT
FEAR

Prelude

If you're looking for a book about courage, fun, excitement, and is very emotionally charged, then here it is. As we all know being ill can be very difficult for adults and especially hard our kids. Some illness can be down right scary and unforgiving to where it makes us seek comfort and understanding of just what it is we have and what our love ones are going through. Cell Mate is written just for those difficult times. It's a realistic, well put together, yet eye-opening story for children battling a terrible disease. It's about how an awful sickness brings two kids and become best friends while fighting cancer in a local cancer treatment hospital. Kids as well as adults will feel connected and walk away with this story in their hearts for years to come. So sit back and get ready for a motivational story that will race it's way right into your hearts and mind.

Cell Mates

On the week of Easter, Ashley, a beautiful eight year old with long red hair, woke up with fever, a bad headache, and very pale skin. But even with not feeling well she still wanted to go to school for the Easter Egg hunt and to make cards for her family and friends.

"Please Mom, can I please go," she asked while starting to cough.

"No baby." said Mr. Wiggins, her dad who stood in the door way, "It's to the hospital for you young lady,"he added.

An hour later they arrived to find out what was making her feel so bad. Blood was drawn and vitals was taken before being taken down the hall to room #5. which was very cold. As the family waited Ashley started throwing up, not once but twice before the nurses came running. Dad held and gently rocked her just before the door opened. It was Dr. Day, a tall thin- middle aged man with papers between his fingers and he wasn't smiling.

"Doc. whats the news," asked dad as he continued to rock.

" Mr. Wiggins can I talk to you and your wife in the hall?"

"Sure."

 Dad laid Ashley on the bed and stepped out the room. Miss. Wiggins followed.

"What is it doctor.?", asked dad.

1

"Well I have bad and good news. Ashley doesn't have enough normal blood cells which means she may have leukemia and if that's true, after more tests then the good news is that we may have caught it early enough to fix it."

"Oh no. You mean my baby may have cancer?," asked Miss Wiggins while holding her husband hand tightly.

"Yes mam, but we wont know for sure until we run more test."

The hall was quiet as the Doc continued to talk.

"So what we want to do, if it's OK with you, is keep her overnight and find out fore sure."

" Yes doctor. Whatever it takes."

"Great! I'll have my nurses get her admitted and taken up stairs,"

"Great," said dad.

Soon as the Wiggins opened the door Ashley set up in bed and asked," Daddy I heard the word leukemia. What is leukemia?" Is that what's wrong with me?"

Surprised, mom and looked at each other and said,"No baby. We're not sure yet. Some more tests have to be done so we can know for-sure."

"But what is Leukemia."

Mom sat beside Ashley and said," You see dear, your body is made up of different types of cells, and these cells have different jobs to do. Like people, these cells must work together to get the job done. But there are some cells that are troublemakers that get in the way of the work that the good cells are doing. Understand?"

"I think so. Is that why I don't feel good? "

"Maybe but we are going to stay here all night until we find out for sure, OK?", said dad.

"Yes sir, but why did I get the mean cells?,"

"Honey don't know why you might have those mean cells, but the doctors will find them and get rid of all the bad ones so you can get better, alright?" said mom.

"Did I do something wrong?"

"No baby. You did nothing wrong," said dad while giving her a big hug. "And there is no need to worry because after we get all the test results back, the doctors and nice nurses will know how to fix whats been bothering my baby girl."

Ashley smiled and gave a big hug back.

About an hour later Ashley was in her room with more blood being drawn. There was another person in the bed next to hers. A colorful divider blocked the view but she could see small house shoes under the bed.

3

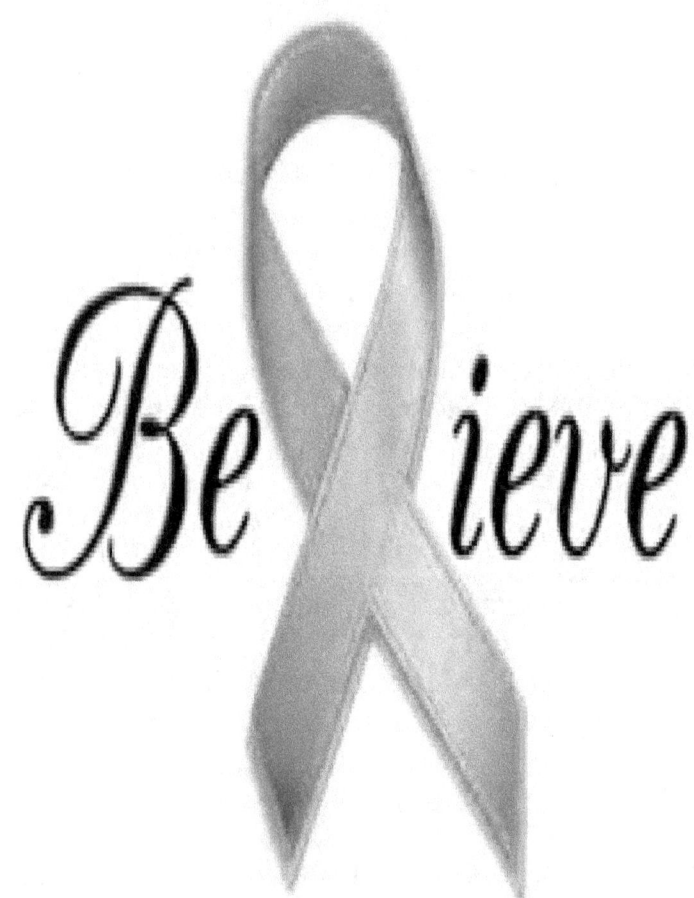

It's now 11:00 and Dad got comfortable in a large chair by the window while mom laid in bed with Ashley. "Good night," they all said.

The next morning mom and dad went down to the cafeteria for breakfast while Ashley rested. But when she woke up a short chubby kid with rosy cheeks and big brown eyes was standing next to her bed, staring quietly.

"Who are you?," asked Ashley while trying to focus on his face.

"I'm Travis but you can call me Hercules"

"Hercules? You don't look like Hercules."

"Not now but I will one day. My dad said if I keep playing football I'm gonna be as strong as my favorite player who really looks like Hercules. Want to see my muscles?"

"No. I want to see my mom and dad."

"Oh I heard them leaving to go eat downstairs but I think they're coming back, at least that's what your mom said."

"Oh.", said Ashley as she began to sat up.

"What's your name?"asked Travis.

"Ashley Renee Wiggins."

"Wow, that's nice."

5

"Why are you in here Travis?"

"Cancer."

"Oh."

What's wrong with you? Why are you here?

Ashley raised here shoulders and said,"I don't know yet. My mom said I might have some bad cells fighting some good cells."

"Oh yea. the doctor said I might have that same thing, but I also have something called a tumor in the back of my head."

"Does it hurt?"

"Sometimes but mostly when I play a lot."

"Are you hurting now?"

"No, but when it does ache sometimes I throw up."

Then they heard Ashley's parents coming up the hall way. Travis said, "Well it was fun talking to you but I'm gonna get back in my bed."

"OK, see-ya later."

And just as Travis laid down the door swung open with her parents standing in front of Dr. Day.

"Well there she is, awake and bright eyed," said the doctor before checking her vitals. "How do you feel today?"

"My head still hurts some."

"Yea and I'm sorry sweetie but now we know whats making you feel that way."said Dr, Day.

Ashley's parents moved closer.

"You young lady have something we call leukemia. And we know just how to fight those bad cells your parents told you about. So there is nothing to worry about, OK sweetie?"

"Yes sir," said Ashley while looking at her dad. She wasn't worried anymore after Dr. Day took his time and explained everything. Then it was time for her parents to leave. This made mom and dad very sad.

After a the treatment plan started Ashley and Travis had become friends. And because the radiation took so much of their energy they had to find fun things to do inside their room until one day, on a Sunday, there was no treatment scheduled. Ashley woke up first feeling better. She noticed on her table a diet food chart showing all types of healthy food they can and should eat.

"Morning Travis," whispered Ashley as she does every day before 8:am. In a low groggy tone Travis answered back,"Morning."

"It's your turn to order breakfast you-know," said Ashley while leaning over her bed. At first she hears nothing so she quietly waits for a answer before pulling her cutely painted feet out from under the covers. "Travis, are you sleeping again?",

"No just thinking." Then he started to smile and asked, "Do you want to have some fun?

"Yea."

"OK, lets sneak down to the kitchen and order our own food like adults."

Excited, Ashley eyes widened before she slid out off the bed, pushed the colorful divider back, and said, " lets do it."

"OK,"

In a rush she put on her robe and pink furry slippers. Travis begin doing the same but with spider man slippers.

"Are you sure about this? I mean, you know we can get into some big trouble," said Ashley.

"Don't worry. We'll be back before you know it." answered Travis while moving towards the door only one slipper on.

"Can you help me find my other house shoe?"

Ashley started giggling and said,"Sure ", and began searching under his bed.

Then, both armed with their IV poles, they eased open the door, looked out, and whispered, "Coast is clear, lets go."

The two nurses at the nurse station was very busy which made it easy to crawl pass the long desk and down the hall to an empty elevator.

Once inside Travis said,"Wow!, that was scary,"

"Sure was ," said Ashley after pushing the up button.

Being only three floors up the ride didn't take long before it was off to the huge kitchen.

Barely seeing over the tray rail they picked what they wanted and headed to checkout but they forgot one thing, they had no money. The thought of paying never crossed their minds because everything was always brought to them.

"That will be $8.67cent please,"said a large middle aged cashier that had seriousness all over her face.

Travis patted his empty robe pockets and looked at Ashley who had just done the same. The kitchen cook and supervisor both made there way over to see what was stopping the line. The closer they got the wider Travis and Ashley eyes got with their hearts beating faster and faster until they grabbed their poles and took off without their food. In front of the elevator they stood, waiting for the doors to open. But the kitchen supervisor was closing in fast.

Ashley nervously whispered, "Please hurry", while reaching for Travis's sweaty hand. And before the supervisor could say "Stop", the doors opened and closed just as they saw him appear.

"Oh man we made it," said Travis with shortness of breath.

"Yea, that was close."
Then Ashley saw Travis go down on one knee.

"What's wrong?," she asked. "Stand up, the doors are about to open."

"Tire, I'm too tired."

But when the doors opened Ashley had his arm around her shoulder and her hand around his waist helping him pack to the room. This time the nurse was doing rounds and just as Ashley helped Travis back into bed, their nurse came in. Travis covered up and played sleep while Ashley started stretching as if she had just woke up. Minutes later the nurse was gone.

"Ashley."

"What?"

I'm still hungry," said Travis while rubbing his stomach.

"Me to but I'm too tired to go back. Think we better wait."

"Yea, guess your right, but I'm still hungry."

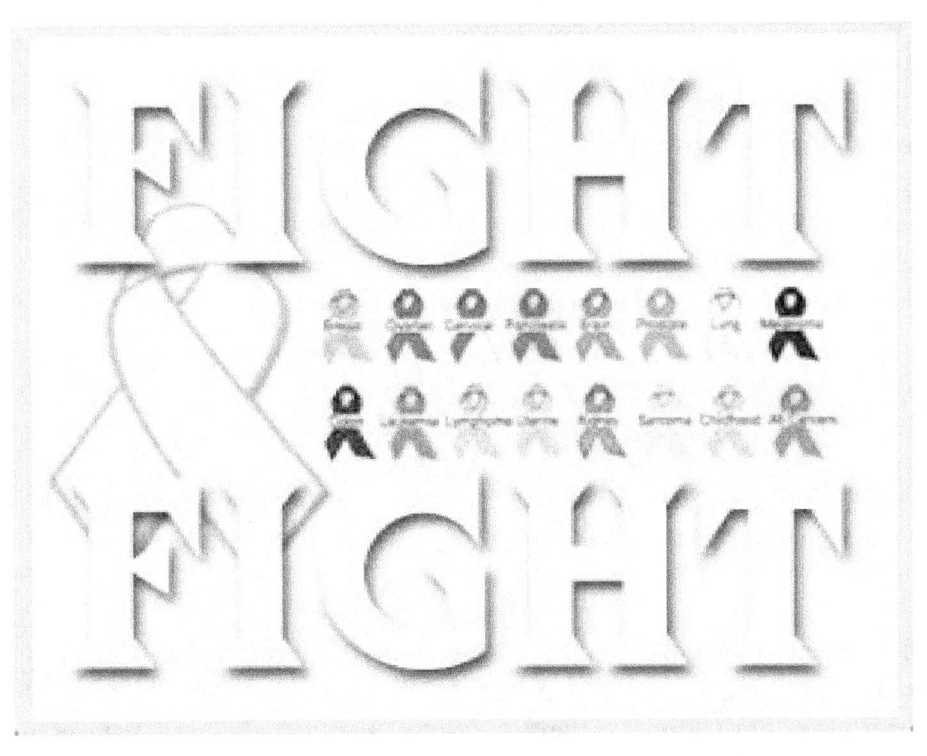

11

"Well don't be looking over here. I'm not a sandwich."

"Hmmmmmm,"said Travis while smiling.

Ashley started laughing before saying, " You better stop it," and throwing her pillow at him.

Then the door opened with the kitchen supervisor walking in. Travis flipped and pretended to be sleep again while Ashley slowly pulled the covers over her nose to where only her eyes could be seen.

"Well well well.", said the every slim but tall visitor. So this is your hideout."

Still not a word was spoken back as the room seemed to get smaller until the door opened again but only this time it opened with the smell of breakfast filling the air.

"Next time no sneaking out to the kitchen. We'll bring it to you along with anything else you may need." said Mr. Henry the kitchen supervisor. "We here at Atlanta Regional Medical Cancer Center wants you two to take it easy, don't worry about nothing, and get better so you can go home."

Travis started to move after hearing the kindness in the supervisors voice and the strong smell of breakfast.

"Yes sir," they both said before digging into their food.

Then Mr. Henry left leaving the room quiet again. Between the scrapping of the forks and spoons against the plates, laughter could be heard in the distance from kids playing outside. Ashley slowly put her spoon down and went to the huge window where she could clearly see across the street onto a school playground. Travis sees his friend staring out, and decides to join her.

"Are you OK?" he asked.

"Yea, just miss playing with my friends," said Ashley while resting her arms on the window seal.

"Me to."

"Did you have lots of friends," asked Ashley without changing position.

Travis didn't answer, dropped his head, and took a deep breath before turning and crawling back into bed.

Ashley was curious and walked over.

"Well?" she asked.

"Well what?"

"You know. Did you have a lot of friends you did stuff with?

While looking away Travis answered, "no"

"Why not?"

13

"Cause."

"Cause what?"

"Cause nothing. What do you care?

"Cause I do?

"Why?"

"Cause I just do and because I'm your friend."

Travis, before turning and facing Ashley, wiped a tear away and said," I don't have any friends and don't have parents. When I got sick with this stupid disease my foster parents brought me here. At first I was getting visits and phone calls but no more."

"Why not?," asked Ashley as she now sat at the end of his bed,

"Because the people that were taking care of me ran out of money and stopped coming, so now it's just been me."

Ashley stared at his quivering lips and said,"And me. You got me silly."

Travis looked up and gave a quick smirk followed by a soft, "thanks." And as she walked back to the window he said, " Don't worry, they will fix us cause if they don't, then I will fix them because I'm Hercules."

14

YOU think YOU'RE tough, I'm gonna beat cancer

Ashley started laughing while focusing her attention back on the other kids. She pressed her hand and forehead against the window and let out a big sigh.

Although there was no treatments scheduled for rest of the day, tomorrow was a biggie for Travis and he knew all about it from his long time case worker who he really liked and trusted. Miss April had been watching over Travis since he first arrived. And took a deep liking to him which always made Travis feel not so alone. So today was a free day. Movies, games, and vital-signs were all they had to look forward to until the evening hours. This is when the doctors make their rounds and talked about whats going to happen the next day. And to answer any and all questions.

By now there were very little they didn't know about each other and when it comes to their illnesses and treatments, everything could be heard past the thin divider. Neither seemed to care nor wanted to hide anything. They were best friends. Then the phone rang with Travis answering but quickly turned it over to Ashley.

"Here, its your mom."

"Oh great, give-me give-me."she said before pacing the floor for about 15 min. then hanging up after a smile and exchanges of, "I love you." Then she shuffled back over to Travis and shared the great news.

"Hey guess what?

"What?," said Travis who sad and wished he had parents to talk to.

"My mom and dad are coming and bringing me a gift. And guess what else?

"What?"

"They are bringing you something to."

Travis quickly set up and asked," What is it?'

"Don't know. She wouldn't say."

"Aaaaawwww man. I bet it's a game or a huge toy," said Travis with joy.

"Not sure but I hope it's good."

Then after 3 or 4 minutes of quiet brainstorming Travis asked, "Do you want to race to the end of the hall and back?"

Na, I'm too tired. Feeling weak again."

"Oh, OK, well good night."

"Good night."

Moments later with all the lights out, Ashley asked,"Do you want to hear a joke my grandpa told me?"

"Sure," whispered Travis with his eyes closed.

"OK, what did the water say to the boat?"

"I don't know."

"Nothing, it just waved."

Immediately Travis started snickering with a loud snorkel. So did Ashley before sharing another one.

"How do you make a tissue dance?

"How?" asked Travis.

"By putting a little bogey in it."

Soon both their laughter became louder with chuckles and coughs. Then Travis said, "Wait I got one. Why did the tomato turn red?"

"I don't know."

"It saw the salad dressing."

The noise became so loud the door swung open with a frowning nurse standing with her hands on her hips.

"OK guys, keep it down. We don't want to wake the others, besides Mr. Travis, you have a big day tomorrow so try and get some rest."

"Yes mam."

And as soon as the nurse walked out low giggles started again and didn't stop until they where sound asleep.

18

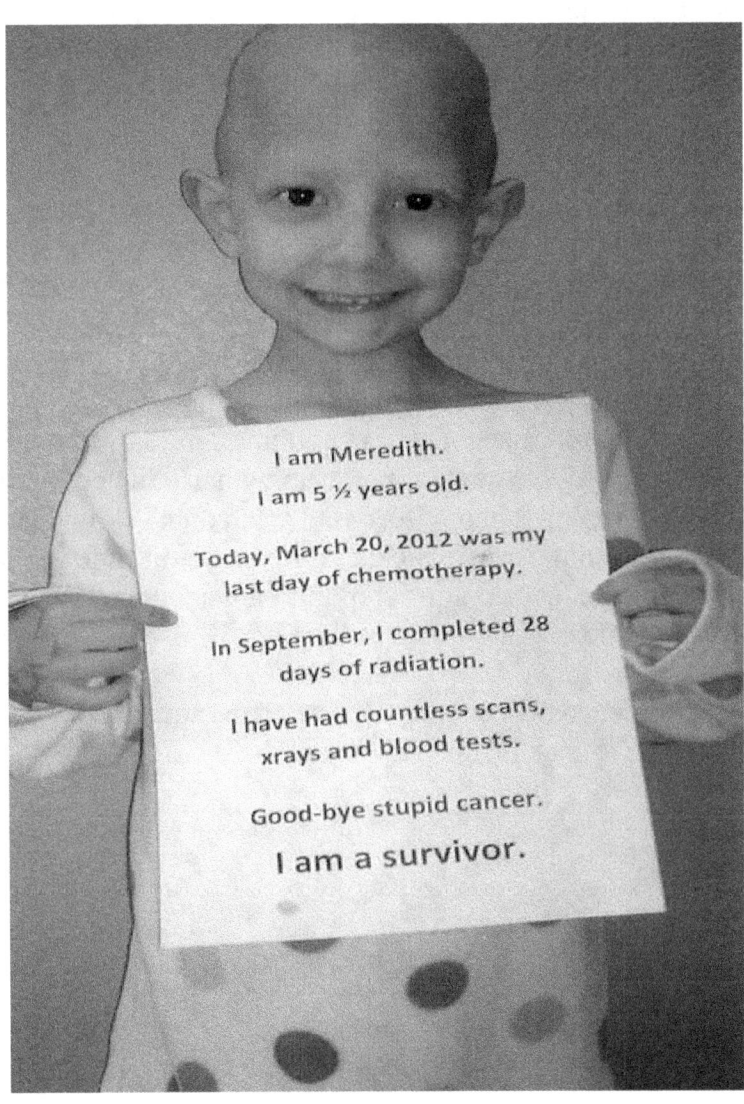

I am Meredith.

I am 5 ½ years old.

Today, March 20, 2012 was my last day of chemotherapy.

In September, I completed 28 days of radiation.

I have had countless scans, xrays and blood tests.

Good-bye stupid cancer.

I am a survivor.

An hour later Travis wakes up, quietly gets out of bed and checks on Ashley like he has been doing every night. He first stares at her to see if shes breathing then makes sure shes covered up before whispering something quickly in her ear. Ashley never moves and he never tells what he says.

The next morning seemed to come faster than normal. The sound of nurses was the first thing heard in the room.

"Morning kiddo, Rise-and-shine,"said Dr. Chow who came in behind the nurses and who was doing the surgery.

Travis was quiet as his doctor explained everything that was about to happen. Ashley could see and hear everything. She saw that he wasn't nervous and gave him a thumbs up with a smile before he was rolled away. Ashley was happy for Travis, and didn't show fear but she was unsure about her own sickness. It was about time for her parents to arrive but she couldn't stop thinking about her friend. Then the nurse and social worker walked in.

Ashley dear how would you like to come to the surgery room with Travis? He just told us that he wants you there."

"He did?'

"Sure did."

"OK, lets go, but first I have to leave a note for my mom and dad. They are coming today."

"Alright then. How about we let them know where you are and bring them too.

"You can do that?," asked Ashley excitedly.

"Sure can, now get dressed so we can hurry."

"Yes mam."

And before Travis went to sleep Ashley walked up and squeezed his hand.

"I thought you weren't coming,"said Travis from behind a oxygen mask. Ashley was too shy and nervous to speak, so she just raised her shoulders and smiled just before it was time. And because the surgery was gonna last a while she was taken back to her room to wait for her parents. Ten minutes later they arrived.

Mom gave hugs first before noticing Travis was gone. She asked," Where is your friend Ashley?"

"In surgery."

"Aaawww, I'm sorry honey. Do you want to talk about it?"

"No, I know he's only getting fixed. But can I be there when he wakes up?"

"We'll have to see."said mom while dad stepped out to ask one of the nurses if it would be OK. The answer made him smile and he couldn't wait to tell the good news. So when he walked back in the room mom was on the bed brushing Ashley's hair.

"How do you feel?," asked dad.

"Tired, but I feel better than yesterday," said Ashley with her head softly laying on mom's chest.

Well that's good. Guess that means the good cell are winning, right?"

"I hope so cause I miss my cat Prince, my room, my friends, and my school."

"Maybe the treatments are working."said mom.

Then Ashley started thinking and said,"Mom can I ask you something?"

"Sure honey, what is it?"

"Can we take Travis home with us when I leave?"

"Oh Ashley," chuckled mom. "He's not like a puppy in a window dear that we can buy and take home. So no honey and I don't think his parents would like us taking their child."

"Yes they would! I mean they wouldn't care."

"What?"

"Yea, because he doesn't have parents anymore. He said," They ran out of money and never came back. They left him here."

"Oh my goodness. How long has he been here?"

"I don't know?"

"Poor thing.", said mom before looking at dad.

"Yea that is pretty sad, but I do have good news,". The nurse gave the OK for you to go visit him."

"Yaaaaaa, can we go now?"

"Nope. She said, "After surgery."

Then mom remember the gifts. "Oh here, look what we got for you."

"Oh goody, what is it?! Let me see."

Mom opened a small pink bag and pulled out a bright red camera.

"WOOOOW," said Ashley with her hands over her mouth.

"You like it?

"Yes mam, Woo-ow! My very first camera. Now I can take lots of pictures.

"Yelp, I think she likes it,"said dad.

23

"Oh thank you mommie".

"And guess what else?" We got your friend a gift to.

"You did?!"

Sure did and we are going to let you give it to him when you see him.

"Oh boy, he's going to love it! Wait, what is it?"

"Same as what you have , but a different color."said mom while pulling it out of a separate bag that has Travis written on it. The first thing Ashley saw was bright blue which made her like it even more.

"He is gonna love it."

Then there was knocking at the door.

"Knock knock," said an odd voice. "Hi, it's Tootles the clown and he's here to give you something." said the nurse.

Ashley hurried and sat on her dads lap waiting for Toddles to do some magic tricks. His first trick had flowers come out of his big hat. Then bubbles, then a stack of playing cards. A colorful ball fell out of his pocket and bounced around, while sprayed Ashley with a water gun. And then he had a baby rabbit pop out.

"Woo ow, that's cool." said Ashley.

Dad asked Toddles," Is there any candy in there?"

"Honey stop."said mom."This is for the kids."

Everyone laughs as Toddles thought for a moment and tapped the hat once more before pulling out a hand full of candy. At that moment dad was as happy as Ashley. After an hour of visiting, the clown waved and left the room. Ashley was so excited that she had forgot all about her friend until another nurse walked in and asked, "Are you ready to go visit your roomy?"

"You betcha,"shouted Ashley.

"OK you guys can follow me," said the smiling nurse as she led the way.

Armed with only Travis's bag of goodies the Wiggins were taken to a small room with light blue walls not far from the OR. Ashley was first to follow the nurse in. They could see Travis laying on his side and not moving so they stayed back.

"OK you only have a few minutes to visit. I'll be back," said the nurse. But before she left she called out to him," Travis ,Travis you have visitors." Ashley moved closer before looking back at mom and dad. Travis opened his eyes and in a soft voice said, "You're here."

"Of-course silly."

This made him smile.

"Here, we have something for you."
25

"What is it?"

Ashley reached in the bag and showed it to him.

"Wow! my own? Cool."

"I have one to."

"Now we can take lots of pictures."

"Yea, that's what I said," said Ashley before asking," Did it hurt?"

"Hurts a little now."

"Did you cry?"

"Nope."

"Was there a lot of blood,?" but before he could answer, Dad said,"Alright Ashley, that's enough questions for now. It's time to go so he can rest."

"Yes sir." Bye Travis, I'll see you later."

"OK."

On the elevator Ashley looked up and asked her dad, "Is he gonna be OK?"

"Sure honey, he's gonna be just fine."

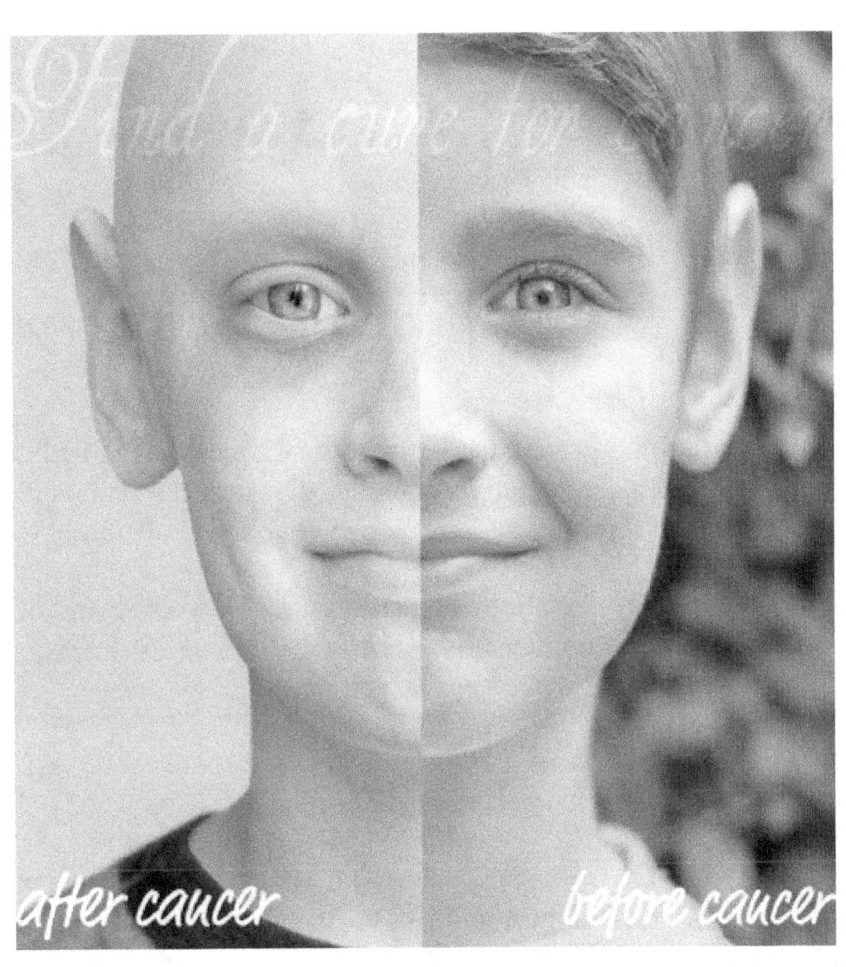

after cancer   before cancer

27

"Are they gonna do the same thing to me?"

"No baby?"

"Hope not cause I would be scared."

"Nothing to fear. These are the best doctors and they will take good care of you."

"I'm tired now. I wanna take a nap."

"OK, we'll get you tucked in before we leave," said mom while picking her up.

And soon after they were back in the room, Ashley was in bed and sound asleep. Mom and Dad left quietly. The next day Travis arrived. He was so excited to see Ashley that he went straight to her.

"How do you feel? Are all the bad stuff gone? Do you get to go home now?," asked Ashley.

"Nope not yet.

"Oh OK,"

And for the next two weeks Travis and Ashley took lots of pictures, played lots of video games, told lots of jokes, sang lots of fun songs, and getting lots of rest until one morning Travis woke up and saw that he was alone. Ashley was gone but he didn't know where.

"Ashley," he called, but there was answer. He slowly gets out of bed and looks in the hallway, still no Ashley. So he climbed back in bed and pushed the call button. A nurse answers.

"May I help you?"

"Yes mam. I can't find my friend."

"Oh she's OK Travis, and will be back anytime now."

"OK."

So while he waited Travis attempted to clean and straighten Ashley's bed before finding an opened diary. As he was about to close it he saw the words "Please God heal me. Help the good cells beat the bad ones so I can be normal again." This made him sad so he closed and covered the book with the large pillow and went back to bed.

An hour later he heard Ashley's voice in the hallway just outside the door. She was holding her moms hand when she came in.

"OK baby, mommy has to go to work now. Are you gonna be OK?,"

"Yes mam."

Mom kissed her on the head and waved at Travis before leaving the room. Travis waited till the door closed and said,"Hey Ashley."

"Hey,"

"Where have you been?"

"Surgery! Why?, What's wrong and what's that thing sticking out of your chest?"

"Still tired Ashley said," It's a port. I have to have chemo."

"What does it do?"

"It's to help kill more of those bad cell and it's there so I don't have to get stuck by needles anymore."

"Woooow!, that's cool. I want one. How much did it cost? I got almost seven dollars in my drawer."

"Don't know. My mom and dad pay for everything."

"Oh probably cost-ed a whole bunch, ha?,"said Travis while leaning in closer for a better look. He also could tell that Ashley was sleepy so he walked to the window , stared out at the playground, and asked," What do you want to be when you grow up?"

Ashley opened her eyes, thought about it, then answered. " A doctor so I can fix people and kill all the bad cells all over the world."

Travis never turned around but said,"I want to be a pro football player and make lots of money so I can help my next family and friends."

" That's nice,"said Ashley before covering up and falling to sleep.

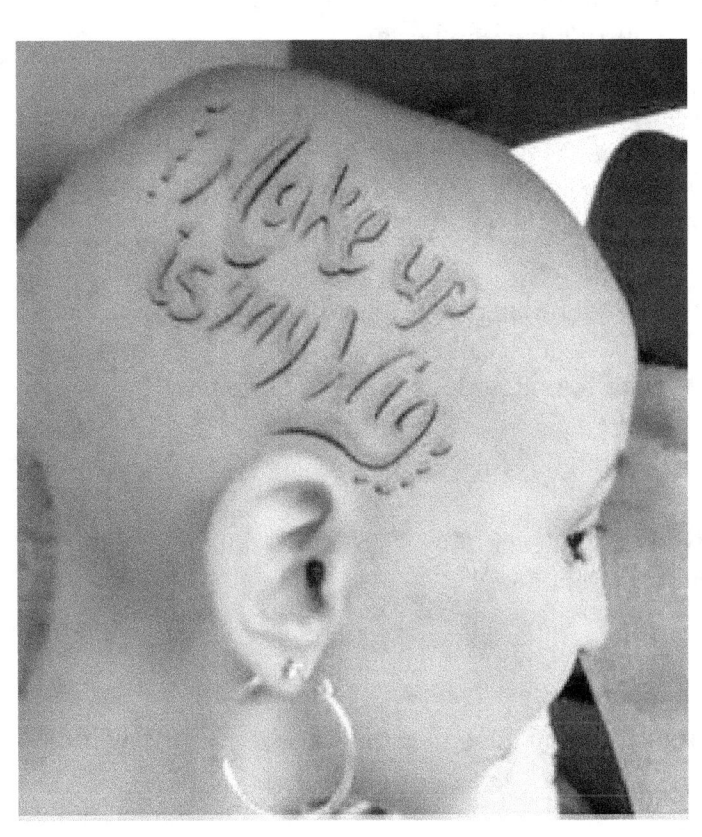

But later that night Ashley woke to drink some water and saw Travis sound asleep. She smiled and had a idea. Quietly she searched her locker and found her large toy spider she named PJ. It was yellow, red, and black with very long and hairy legs. It looked very real. Slowly she tip-toes over and carefully puts PJ on top of Travis's covers then hurried back to her bed.

Two hours later she and Travis were suddenly awaken by a nurse who came in and saw the spider which made her start screaming, jumping, and pointing. Travis sees it and starts screaming as well before pulling the covers over his head.

Ashley couldn't stop laughing until she saw the frowning nurse holding the spider and walking towards her. The room got quiet as the nurse spoke," Ashley does this belong to you?"

"Yes mam,"

"Look sweetie, you can't play games like this in the hospital. People can get hurt, understand?"

Ashley answered with her head down,"Yes mam.'

"And I'm gonna keep the spider with me for a little while, OK?"

OK."

After she walks out Travis slowly peaks out from under the covers, looks at Ashley, and they both started laughing. For the rest of the day they laughed and talked about what the nurse did and watched movies until bed time.

A week later, while watching her favorite cartoons, Ashley notices lots of hair in her comb and on her pillow. "Oh no, oh no", she called her mom while Travis called for the nurse. Her eyes filled with tears as she waited for her mom to answer.

"Mom, my hair is coming out."

"What? Oh baby mommie will be right there,OK . Don't worry."

The door opened just as Ashley put the phone down.

"Whats going on? Why are you upset Ashley?" asked the nurse.

"My hair, my hair wont stop coming out! Why wont it stop!?"she cried.

"Oh sweetie I'm sorry", said the nurse while hugging Ashley tightly. "Listen do you remember what the doctor said about side effects?"

"Yes."

"Good because this is one of them. You see Ashley this kind of medicine causes stuff like this to happen but it also does good things to help people like kill all those bad cells, understand?"

Yes mam."

A little while later mom and dad walked in with all their hair cut off and carrying a small white bag. Ashley was shocked but rushes over and jumps into her daddy's arms with water eyes.

"Hey, there's my beautiful little girl. Guess what we have for you."

She wipes her face, looks in, and sees five bright color scarfs. There was a red one, a pink one, a blue one, a white, and a black one. Ashley chose the red one, which is her favorite color, and let mom put it on her. And to make her feel better dad put on the blue one while mom tied the white on her head. Doing all of this made really made Ashley feel better to where she started smiling again.

Later that night, just before bed, Travis walks over to Ashley and says, " I'm sorry about what happened to you today."
Ashley smiled and pulled out the black scarf.

"Would you like to wear this one?"

Surprised he said, " Sure!"and quickly put it on.

"That looks cool on you,".

"Thanks, yours to? I better go to bed now. Goodnight."

"Goodnight,"said Ashley before turning off her light.

And after a few more weeks of treatment it was time for both to leave. Ashley was still weak but was ready to go. The doctor said almost all the bad cells was gone and the rest was going to die later. Then they gave a bag of medications to take home, in-order to kill the rest of the bad cells. She was so happy that she hugged the doctor and nurses before giving Travis a hug. The next morning mom and dad came and were ready to take Ashley back home.

Travis sat quietly watching Ashley pack up all her stuff. He too was finished with his treatments but had no home to go to. He was loosing his best friend until Mr. Wiggins said, " Well Travis what are you waiting on, pack your stuff. You're going home with us."

Instantly the room got quiet and Ashley dropped her bags. Neither she nor Travis could believe their ears.

"Mom is it true or is daddy playing? Travis can come home with us?"

Smiling mom nodded her head as dad said, " Yes it is. We did all the paper work a few weeks ago and wanted it to be a surprise."

Travis slowly walked over with his hands covering his face.

"It's OK son, don't cry. Everything is gonna be alright now, said dad before gently picking him up. Then mom and Ashley came over and also gave Travis a big hug.

"I love you Travis,"said Ashley.

"Love you to."

"I know. You tell me every night.

"You mean you were awake?"

"Hah aha, yelp, sure was."

THE END
35

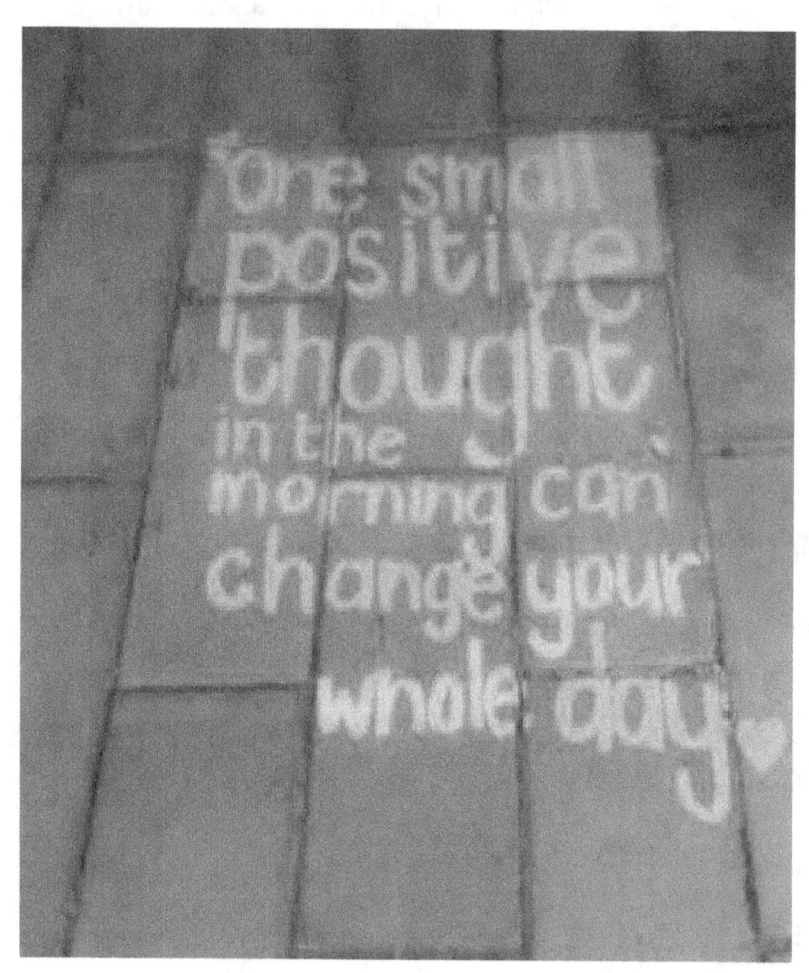

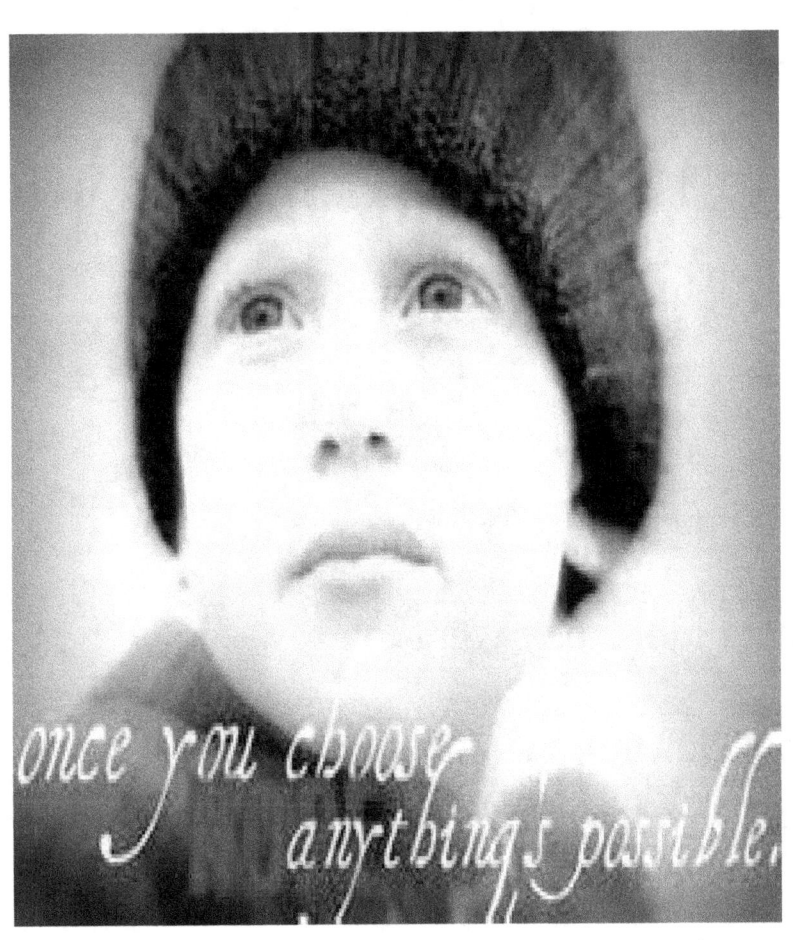

once you choose anything's possible.

Questions

Who had the tumor in their head?

_____

What illness did the doctor say the girl had?

_____

Who couldn't find their slipper?

_____

What color scarf did the girl wear?

_____

Who had no family?

_____

What did the boy want to grow up and be?

_____

What was mom and dads last name?

_____

What does Leukemia means?

_____

What was the gift mom and dad bought?

_____

What medicine made the girls hair come out?

_____

What was the big surprise at the end of the story?

_____

What was the port used for?

_____

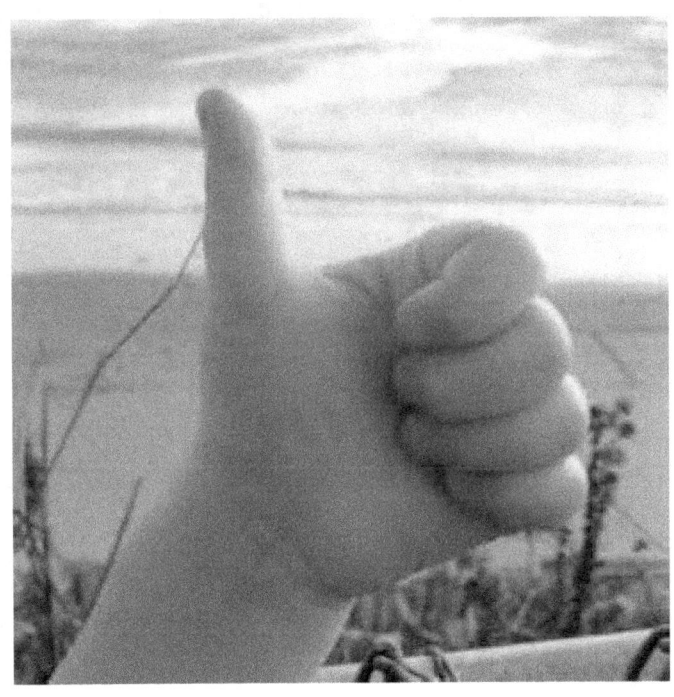

LETS FIGHT
BY EATING
RIGHT

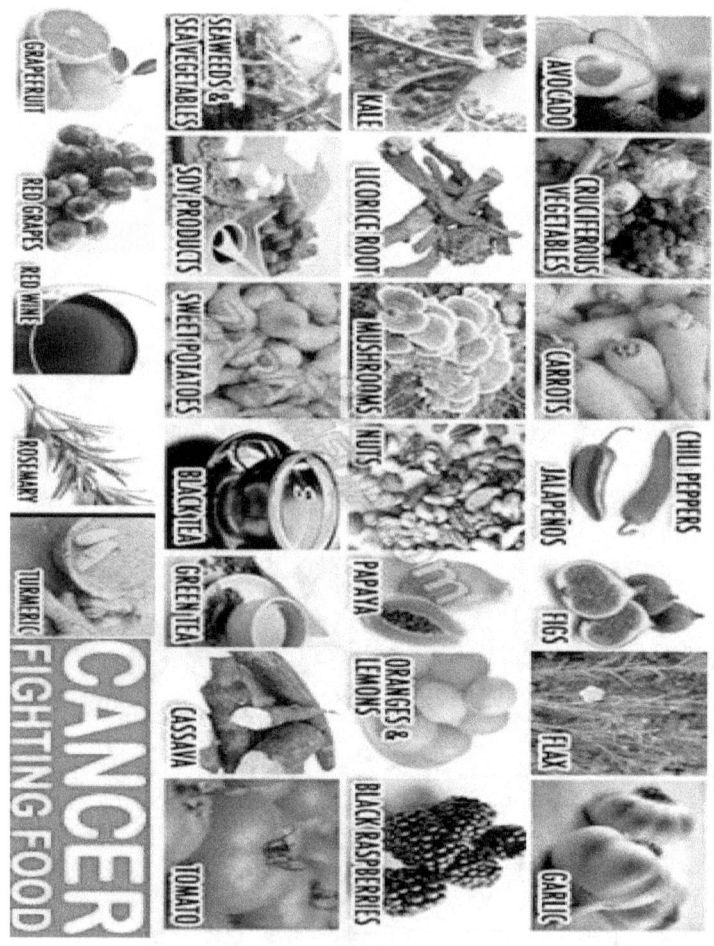

Cancer Fighting Foods

Green tea
Blackberries
Blueberries
Lemon
Apples
Kale
Ginseng

Ginger
Turmeric
Cinnamon
Artichokes
Garlic
Tomato
Olive oil

Pomegranate
Green leafy-vegetables
Cauliflower
Avocado
Nuts & Seeds
Broccoli
Mushrooms

WWW.PLANETAYURVEDA.COM

EATING HEALTHY

YOU ARE STILL
BEAUTIFUL
WITH CANCER

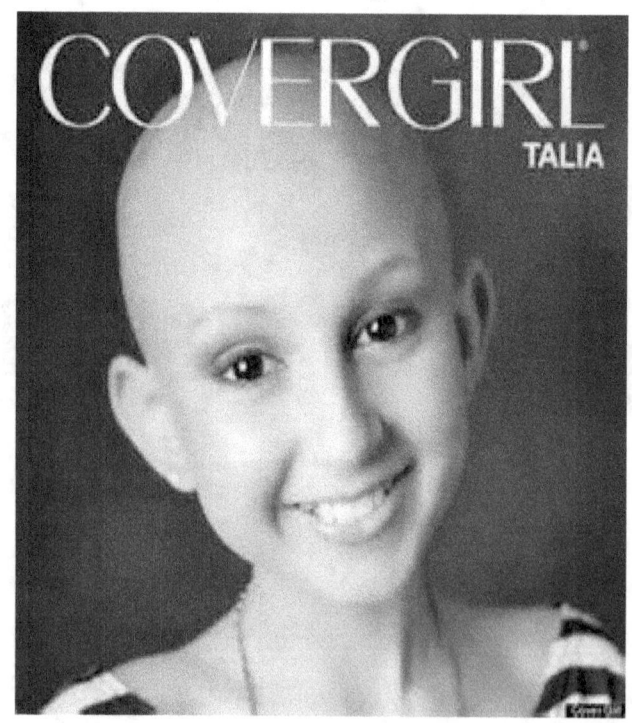

Hang In There
Like Me

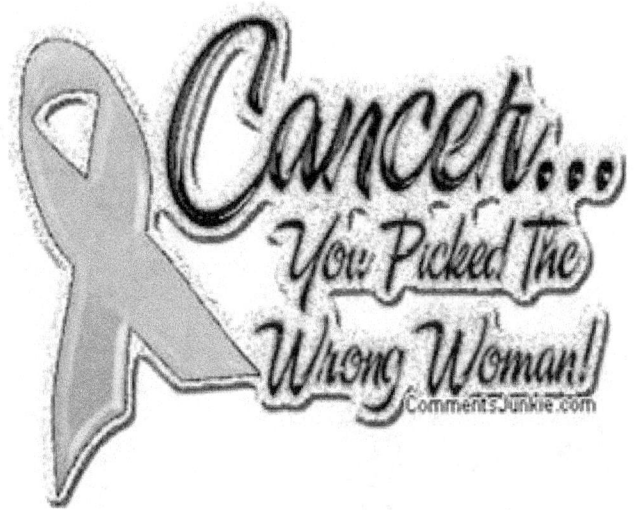

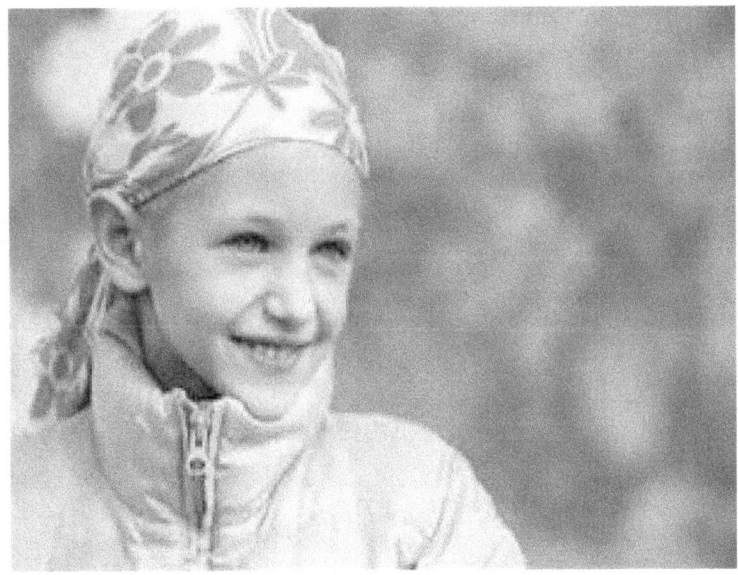

WORD FROM THE AUTHOR

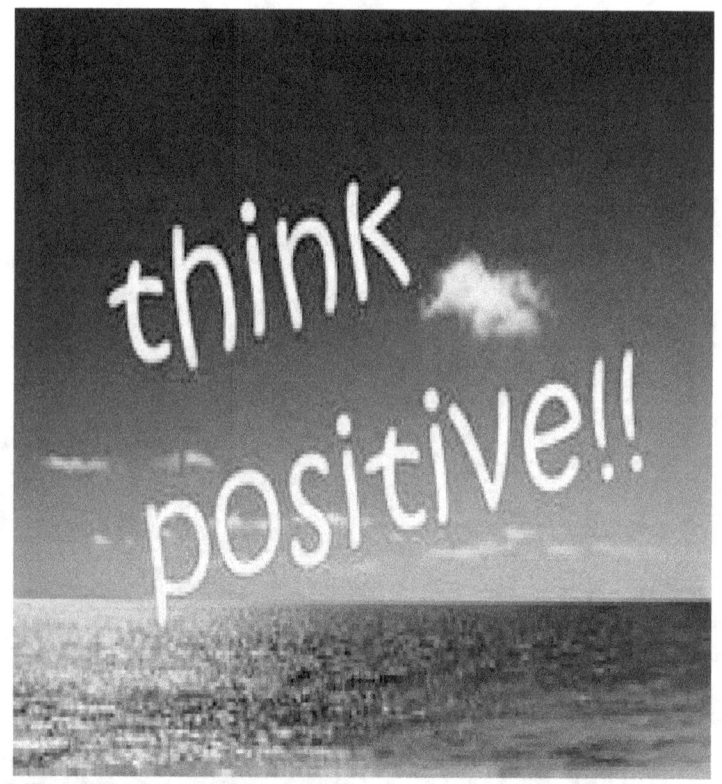

…...AND NEVER LOSS HOPE. LETS FIGHT OUR CANCER TOGETHER

BOOK SIGNING

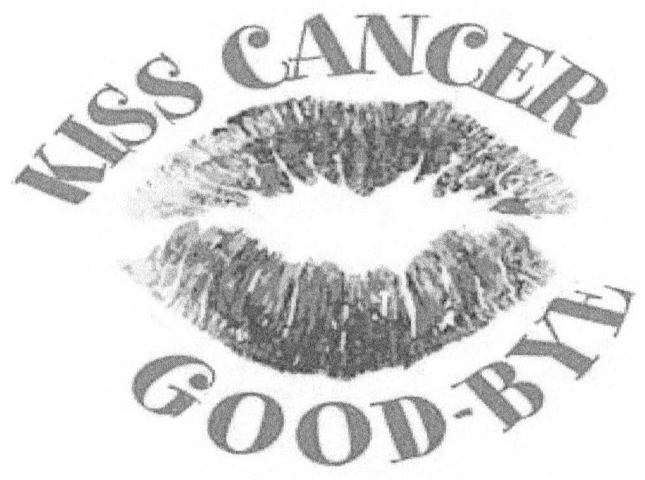

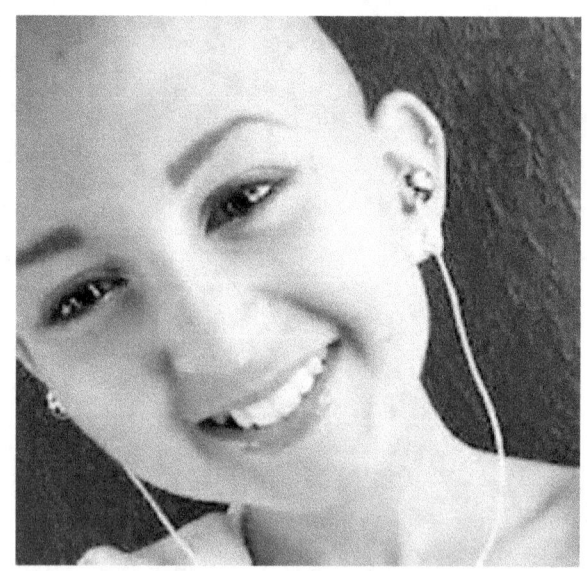

DAIRY

ALBUMS

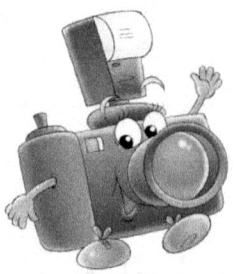

more pictures

Fantastic Resources

These online groups are available 24/7 and most offer chat rooms or discussion boards for patients and families affected by cancer.

- The American Cancer Society has a list of online cancer support resources, including the Cancer Survivors Network, which offers online peer support, chats, discussion boards and other resources for and by people who have been affected by cancer.
- The Livestrong Foundation offers a number of online cancer support resources. The Live strong Cancer Navigation Services provides a host of free services to cancer patients, including helping patients with health insurance issues, finding clinical trials and treatment concerns.
- The Association of Cancer Online Resources (ACOR) offers 142 free online communities for parents, caregivers, family members, and friends to discuss clinical and nonclinical issues and advances pertaining to all forms of a specific disease.
- IHadCancer.com is a peer-to-peer online support resource started by Mailet Lopez, a breast cancer survivor, in 2008. It is a social network that has grown considerably in the last few years, and offers a section in which users can post messages "to cancer."

More Support Groups

- ADEN-CYST - Adenoid Cystic Carcinomas Electronic Support Group (ACOR)
- ALL-L - Adult Acute Lymphocytic Leukemia Email List (ACOR)
- Alliance for Lung Cancer Advocacy, Support, and Education (USA) a non-profit organization aiming to help people with lung cancer through advocacy, psychosocial support programs, and education about the disease and treatment. The site includes sections about lung cancer, symptom management etc.
- Alliance of Genetic Support Groups, Inc A non-profit organization founded in 1986;a national coalition of consumers, professionals and genetic support groups. The site includes details of AGSG, a Directory of Genetic Organizations, resources, on-line newsletter, publications etc.
- American Brain Tumour Association (USA) A non-profit organization founded in 1973 dedicated to the elimination of brain tumors through research and patient education services.
- American Cancer Society (USA) A non-profit organization with over 3400 offices located in all 50 states, plus Puerto Rico. The site has information for both the public and health professionals including information about ACS programs, specific cancers, local branch details etc.
- Aplastic Anaemia Trust, The (UK) The Trust, formerly known as the Marrow Environment Fund was founded in 1985. It is involved in research and support for a plastic anemia (AA) and related diseases. The Web site includes information about AA, support group, fund-raising etc.
- Aplastic Anemia and MDS International Foundation, Inc. This organization, formerly know as A plastic Anemia Foundation of America was founded in 1983. It provides a resource directory for patient assistance, produces educational material and supports research into AA and MDS.
- BLADDER-ONC - Bladder Cancer and Transitional Cell Carcinomas Electronic Support Group

(ACOR)
- Bone Marrow Transplant Support Group (Ireland) Funded in 1994 to provide support for Bone Marrow Transplant patients and their families. The web site includes information, links and the groups Newsletter.
- Brain Tumor Foundation of Canada A national, not-for-profit organization, founded in 1982 to provide support to people affected by brain tumors. The Web site has both English and French language pages which provide details of the organization, its services, events, collaborations.
- Brain Tumor Society (USA) Resources for both patients, relatives, and health professionals
- Bray Cancer Support Centre (Ireland) a non-profit voluntary service founded in 1990 to offer emotional support and practical help to people who had or have cancer and their families and friends. The page includes details of the Drop-in Center and various support groups.
- Cancer Black Care (UK) This is a charity, founded in 1995, which aims to address the cultural and emotional needs of black people affected by cancer. The site includes details of information, support, and advocacy services, contact lists etc.
- Cancer Care Society (UK) A registered charity with branches in various parts of England and Wales providing counseling and support for patients, family and friends.
- Cancer Care, Inc (USA) a national voluntary social service agency, facilities include a toll free telephone helpline. The web site includes details of programs, information about specific cancers and topics including free access to audio clips of teleconferences etc.
- Cancer Plus - Parent's support group (Ireland) a national support group for parents who have a child who has been diagnosed and treated for cancer. This page provides a brief overview of cancer-plus and is located on the Irish Cancer Society web page.
- Cancer Relief Macmillan Fund (UK) National charity, devoted to ensuring the best possible quality of life for people with cancer and supporting over 1,400 Macmillan nurses.
- Cancer Support Association (Australia) CSA is a non-profit support group formed in 1984 by patients and relatives. This site gives details of the organization, 24 hour telephone help-line, meetings, programs etc.
- Cancerkin Centre (Royal Free Hospital, London, UK) a hospital based breast cancer support organization founded in 1987. The organization provide support and rehabilitation programmes and run a specialist Lymphoedema clinic.
- Candlelighters Childhood Cancer Foundation (USA) The CCCF is a non-profit organization which aims to educate, support, serve, and advocate for families of children with cancer, survivors, and health professionals. CCCF was founded in 1970 now has over 43,000 members worldwide.
- Candlelighters Childhood Cancer Foundation of Canada (Canada) This site provides details about the foundation and includes a comprehensive resource center with details of booklets, videos, and other support material.
- CanTeen (Australia) A national support group founded in 1985 by teenagers It provides support for teenagers and young adults (ages 12-24 yrs) living with cancer and their teenage brothers and sisters. The website includes details of pro grammes etc.
- CanTeen - support group (Ireland) A support group for young people with cancer, their brothers, sisters and friends - ages 12 to 20. This page is on the Irish Cancer Society Web site.
- CARCINOID - Carcinoid Cancer Online Support Group Email list
- Children's Brain Tumor Foundation (USA) The CBTF is a non-profit organization founded by families, friends and physicians of children with brain tumors; the foundation raises funds for research. This site includes details of services and events, and articles about brain tumors
- Children's Hospice International A non-profit organization founded in 1983 to provide a

network of support and care for children with life-threatening conditions and their families.
- Children's Leukemia Foundation of Michigan (USA) CLF was founded by parents in 1952 and aims to provide compassionate personalized support for both children and adults with leukemia and other blood disorders. The site includes information about services, Q&A, events, newsletter etc.
- Children's Neuroblastoma Cancer Foundation A non-profit organization providing support, advocacy and funding medical research projects on neuroblastoma. CNCF is based in Bloomingdale, IL, the Web site includes information about the organization, news, events, donations and resources.
- CLL - Chronic Lymphocytic Leukemia Support Group Email List
- Colostomy Care Group (Ireland) support to patients who are about to have or who have had surgery to treat cancer of the colon or rectum. This page is on the Irish Cancer Society web site.
- Corporate Angel Network (USA) Non-profit organization that provides free air transportation to and from recognized US cancer hospitals without regard to their financial resources. The network has helped over 10,000 patients since 1981.
- CTCL-MF - Information and Support for: Cutaneous T-Cell Lymphoma / Mycosis Fungoides Email List
- E-SARCOMA Email List - The Ewing Sarcoma Online Support Group (ACOR) includes details of how to join the list - E-SARCOMA@listserv.acor.org
- EMOTIONAL SUPPORT LIST An general index of Email support lists - including some cancer related.
- Families of Children with Cancer (Toronto, Canada) a registered charity run by volunteers to provide education, support and advocacy for families affected by childhood cancer. FCC is linked with Toronto Hospital for Sick Children, the site has details of FCC, newsletter, library etc
- Foundation for the Children's Oncology Group (formerly the National Childhood Cancer Foundation) (USA) The FCOG is a non-profit organization which supports pediatric cancer treatment and research projects in association with The Children Oncology Group (COG). This site includes information, inspiring stories, news, and links to WWW resources.
- Fountain Centre, The A charitable trust which is attached to the St. Luke's Cancer Wing at The Royal Surrey County Hospital in Guild-ford. It provides counseling, complementary therapies, information and support for patients and their families.
- Francoise Babet Leukaemia Foundation Inc. (Australia) a registered charity since 1995 which provides help and support to patients and families affected by leukemia and other blood disorders. Also provide accommodation and support to overseas patients who are being treated in Oz.
- Give Hope (UK) a national brain tumor organization aiming to provide support and promote awareness and research. The site includes a newsletter, list of events, list of UK addresses, links, and other information.
- (NEW) Hammer Out A Bristol based charity founded in 2002 for the relief, assistance and support of people with brain tumors together with their family and carers. The Web site includes news, details of support group meetings and other events.
- Healthy Young Attitude A group founded in Silicon Valley in 1997 to provide support and information to young adults with cancer. The Web site includes news and events, a bulletin board, information for carers, personal stories, and other resources.
- (NEW) HER2 Support Group.org A non-profit organization which aims to help members by supporting concerns and by providing links to news and current research. The site includes a

message board and details of clinical trials.

- Histiocyte Society Hosted at The Texas Children's Cancer Center and Hematology Service this Web site provides details about the Historicity Society, information about histiocytosis etc.
- Hobart Cancer Support Group An Australian support group for people with cancer and their families
- HUG Hodgkins United Group (Ireland) a support group for patients with Hodgkin's and Non-Hodgkins Lymphomas, their relatives and friends. This page is on the Irish Cancer Society web site.
- Intercultural Cancer Council (USA) The ICC aims to promote policies to improve care and treatment in minorities and medically undeserved cancer patients.
- International Myeloma Foundation This site contains details of the IMF, telephone hotline, and information packs. Online resources include a newsletter, email discussion group, and patient handbook. Also there is information for researchers: grant applications etc.
- Italian Federation of Pediatric Oncology Parent Associations (Home page in English language) The federation was founded in 1995 and brought together 20 Parents Associations involved in support for childhood cancer.
- Jeffrey's Folks Cancer Link (Canada) Jeffery's Folks is a support group for families touched by childhood cancer. The site includes a quarterly newsletter which is part-funded by the Canadian Cancer Society.
- Josep Carreras International Leukaemia Foundation Spanish and English language support. JCILF was founded in 1988 at the behest of the tenor Joseph Carr-eras, and funds leukemia research and the Red-mo register of marrow donors. Details of the foundation and grant applications.
- KIDNEY-ONC - Kidney Cancer Online Support Group Email discussion list
- KIDSCOPE Support organization to help the families and children of cancer patients
- L-M-SARCOMA - Leiomyosarcoma Electronic Support Group Email discussion list
- Let's Face It (UK) A support network for facial disfigured, with worldwide contacts. Founded in 1984 by a patient who had a rare facial cancer.
- Leukaemia Care Society (UK) A support group established in 1967 which provides support for children and adults with leukemia and their families. The web site includes detailed information about the Society and its pro grammes, medical overview and related links.
- Leukaemia Research Fund (UK) A national cancer charity funding research into leukemia and other types of cancer. The site includes online patient information booklets, and research abstracts.
- Leukemia and Lymphoma Society (USA) a national voluntary health agency dedicated to curing leukemia, lymphoma, multiple melanoma, and Hodgkin disease. The web site includes details of the 58 chapters of the society, information booklets, patient services, research etc.
- LIVER-ONC - Liver Cancer Electronic Support Group Email discussion list
- LUNG-ONC - Lung Cancers Internet Support Group Email discussion list
- Lymphoma Association (UK) The association provide emotional support and information to people with lymphatic cancer and to their families, carers and friends. The site has details of the national network of support groups, telephone helpline, online-booklets etc.
- Mary-Helen Mautner Project for Lesbians with Cancer (USA) a tax exempt organization providing education and advocacy for lesbians with cancer and their partners.
- MEL-L Melanoma Support Group (ACOR) Email discussion list
- Men Against Cancer (Ireland) a cancer support group which provides information, advice and support to men who have received a recent diagnosis of prostate or testicular cancer. This page

is on the Irish Cancer Society web site.

- Michael Brandon Young Childhood Cancer Foundation, Inc (USA) MBYCCF is a non-profit organization which provides educational and financial support to children with cancer and their families. It is linked with Pediatric Hematology/Oncology at Duke University and Egleston Children s hospital at Emory.
- Mind over Matter - Testicular Cancer Support Group (UK) a group aiming to provide to support through befriending and to increase awareness of testicular cancer
- Miracle House - NY (USA) a non-profit organization, founded in 1990, which provides accommodation and support to family and friends traveling to visit people with cancer and AIDS who are being treated in New York.
- National Association of Psychological Assistance for Cancer Patients (Turin, Italy) Association National Assistance Psychological Ambulation Cancer is a voluntary service founded in 1980 that offers free psychological help to people with cancer. Italian language with some English support.
- National Children's Cancer Society (USA) NCCS is a non-profit organization founded in 1987 which provides direct financial support to children (to age 18) with cancer and their families. The site includes details of the NCCS International Program, events, services and donations.
- Neurofibromatosis A support page for people affected by Neurofibromatosis
- NHL - Non Hodgkins Lymphoma Support Group Email discussion list
- Norwegian Cancer Society - Den Norske Kreftforening NCS is a national voluntary organization with over 170,000 members. The Web site provides details of the society including member organizations, research, patient support, and international activities. It includes English language pages.
- Oesophageal Patients Association An organization and charity founded in 1985 by survivors of esophageal cancer.
- Ovacome (UK) A national support group for all those concerned with ovarian cancer, involving sufferers, families, friends, carers and health professionals.
- PANCREAS-ONC - Pancreatic Cancer Electronic Support Group Email discussion list
- Patient Advocate Foundation (USA) PAF is a non-profit organization committed to offering support to cancer patients through legislative reform eg. requiring insurers to offer coverage for high dose chemotherapy / ABMT.
- PED-ONC Email List - The Pediatric Cancers Electronic Support Group (ACOR) an moderated discussion list for patients, family, friends, researchers, and physicians to discuss clinical and non-clinical issues relating to childhood cancer. This page includes details about how to subscribe. PED-ONC@MEDINFO.ORG
- Prostate Cancer Charity (UK) A charity launched in 1996 to increase awareness provide support and fund research into prostate cancer, with 12,000 new patients being diagnosed each year in the UK. The site includes information about the prostate, cancer, treatments, FAQ etc
- Prostate Help Assocaition (UK) A support group for all types of prostate problems including prostate cancer.
- Questions and Answers About Finding Cancer Support Groups (Cancer Net) Fact Sheet. General introduction about the role of cancer support groups and how to find them.
- Reach to Recovery - Breast Cancer support group (Ireland) a national support pro-gramme for women who are about to have, or who have recently had breast surgery. This page is on the Irish Cancer Society web site.
- Ron Smith Cancer Appeal (Wales) The appeal has successfully campaigned for a cancer treatment center in North Wales and is raising money for equipment etc. The site is in both

English and Welsh language.
- Scottish Association of Prostate Cancer Support Groups (Scotland, UK) the association was founded by prostate cancer patients and their families in April 1999 to a network of regional support groups and raise awareness of prostate cancer. Registered Scottish charity No.029158.
- Selp-Help and Support Groups - Patient Information Publications (UK) This site includes an index of UK links to health related self-help and support groups sorted by disease type / medical topic. There is a page of links to cancer related support groups in the UK.
- Support for People with Oral and Head and Neck Cancer (SPOHNC) (USA) a not-for-profit organization founded in 1991. SPOHNC provides for the emotional, psychological and humanistic needs of the oral and head and neck cancer. Members can subscribe to a regular Newsletter.
- Support Groups - Menu (OncoLink)
- Tak Tent - Cancer Support Scotland The Web site includes details of Tak Tent support groups throughout Scotland, counseling services, and other Tak Tent projects.
- TC-NET - Testicular Cancer Online Support Group Email discussion list
- Teenage Oncology Patient Support (TOPS) (UK) TOPS is a free club, based in the South West of England, for people aged 12 21 who have, or have had, cancer or leukemia. The Web pages are hosted on the CLIC site and include details of TOPS events and activities.
- The Compassionate Friends - Atlanta Chapters (USA) This site provides support for those suffering bereavement, and is a collaboration of the TCF chapters in Atlanta.
- ThyCa: Thyroid Cancer Survivors' Association A non-profit organization founded in 1995 developing programs to link survivors and healthcare professionals around the world. The web site includes news for survivors about on-line chats, conference, mailing lists and local support groups.
- THYROID-ONC - Thyroid Tumors Electronic Support Group Email discussion list
- UK Brain Tumour Society UKBTS is a registered charity, founded in 1997 by patients, relatives and three charities to provide support, increase awareness and promote research. The Web site includes
- Ulman Fund - for young adults affected by cancer (USA) A non-profit organization founded in 1996 by a cancer survivor. The fund supports young adults affected by cancer and the web site includes details of the Fund, its programs, a guide book, scholarship information, survivors network and links.
- US TOO International, Inc. An independent network of support groups for men with prostate cancer and their families, founded in 1990. The site includes listings of support groups, medical information, events etc with input from a Medical Advisory Board.
- WARMNET - MD Anderson Support Mailing List (ACOR)
- Why me - Helping Children with Cancer (USA) Worcester based non-profit organization that provides emotional and financial support to area children with cancer and their families. This site provides details of the organization, its fund-raising events, support program, and links.
- Young Adults Living With Cancer (USA) An organization dedicated to helping make resources available to young adults who have or have had cancer. "We realize that the conic

There is a 'can' in

Can**cer**

because we CAN beat it!

www.ingramcontent.com/pod-product-compliance
Lightning Source LLC
Chambersburg PA
CBHW060219290526
45789CB00003B/1335